Air Frying for Diabetic Living

Delicious Recipes to Manage your Blood Sugar

Shauve Rivk

Copyright © 2024 by Shauve Rivk

All rights reserved. No part of this book may be reproduced in any form or by any electronic or mechanical means, including information, storage and retrieval systems, without permission in writing from the author, except by a reviewer who may quote brief passages in a review.

Table of Contents

Introduction

Join us as we explore the amazing world of air frying, a game changer for diabetics, in our hunt for a better and more active lifestyle. Can diabetics benefit from air frying?

In this book, we'll look at the special advantages of air-frying for diabetics. Learn how this strategy may help you balance your blood sugar levels while keeping the delicious texture and taste of your favorite dishes.

We will dig into the science of air frying and illustrate how it corresponds with diabetic-friendly diet guidelines, measuring the impact on blood glucose levels.

When it comes to treating diabetes, knowledge is power. Here we look at some of the ways that various cooking techniques could impact blood sugar levels. You may increase your general health by studying the ins and outs of air-frying and then putting that knowledge into practice.

Beginning your air-frying voyage needs a few fundamental principles and activities. These ideas will not only enhance your cooking talents but will also make it simpler to prepare scrumptious, blood sugar-friendly meals.

As we begin on this delightful adventure, allow the enticing smells and healthy ingredients to transform your image of diabetic-friendly cooking.

This is more than merely a cookbook; it's a guide for changing your kitchen into a paradise of health and joy. Prepare to experience the miracle of air frying as we prepare a range of scrumptious delicacies to satisfy your taste buds and assist your diabetic lifestyle.

Let the journey begin!

Why Air Frying for Diabetics?

Beginning a culinary journey suited to the requirements of those managing diabetes involves a thoughtful approach to food preparation.

1. **Healthier Cooking with Less Oil:** Traditional frying techniques can entail soaking food in enormous quantities of oil, which adds additional calories and saturated fats.

Air frying, on the other hand, employs hot air circulation to obtain the necessary crispy texture without the use of excessive oil. This not only minimizes the calorie content of your meals, but it also coincides with the heart-healthy principles essential for diabetes.

2. **Retained Nutrient Value:** One of the biggest concerns for diabetes patients is maintaining a nutrient-dense diet. Conventional cooking procedures, notably boiling and overcooking, could contribute to nutritional loss.

Air-frying excels at retaining the natural quality of meals and sealing in vitamins and minerals that are required for general wellbeing. This makes each meal not only tasty but also nutritionally helpful to your health.

3. **Blood Sugar-Friendly Crunchy Goodness:** While appetites for crunchy and rich textures are universal, people with diabetes must find a balance between pleasure and health. Air-frying

offers the answer by producing the necessary crisp without the downsides of deep-frying. What was the result? Enjoyable, guilt-free meals that avoid blood sugar spikes.

4. **Versatility in Recipe Modification:** Adapting meals to satisfy dietary limits may often feel restrictive. However, air-frying brings up a whole new set of options.

From appetizers to sweets, this approach enables you to replicate a broad variety of foods with diabetic-friendly changes. Enjoy the joys of culinary inventiveness without sacrificing your health.

5. **Time-Efficient and Convenient:** Modern living frequently requires kitchen efficiency while retaining food quality. Air-frying is a time-saving culinary miracle that takes less preheating and cooking time than traditional techniques.

Say goodbye to long cooking periods while retaining the quality of your cuisine.

We urge you to experience the immense advantages of air frying while rethinking the junction of health-conscious eating and culinary delight. Through this culinary approach, we seek to empower you to make educated and savory choices, ensuring that your diabetes journey is not only manageable but also full of exquisite moments of delight. Discover the transforming power of air frying and embark on a culinary journey in which health and flavor coexist.

Understanding the Impact on Blood Sugar

We must evaluate how our dietary choices impact our blood sugar levels on a regular basis.

1. **Glycemic Index and Cooking Techniques:** The glycemic index (GI) assesses how rapidly carbohydrates in a diet elevate blood sugar levels. Different cooking processes may alter a meal's glycemic reactivity.

When we fry products in oil or cook them at high temperatures, the glycemic index rises. Air frying, with its reduced oil content and softer cooking process, promotes a more constant glycemic response, making it an enticing alternative for individuals attempting to regulate blood sugar levels correctly.

2. **Retaining Dietary Fiber:** Dietary fiber has a significant function in delaying sugar absorption and maintaining stable blood glucose levels. Traditional frying processes may result in fiber loss, particularly when breading or coating is applied. Air-frying minimizes this loss, enabling the fiber content of meals to be better retained. This not only supports digestive health but also facilitates the slow release of sugar into the circulation.

3. **The Effect of Cooking Oils on Blood Sugar:** The sort and amount of cooking oil used may drastically influence the glycemic response of a meal. Deep frying, for example, includes extensive oil absorption, which leads to a larger caloric content and resultant blood sugar spikes.

Air-frying utilizes less oil, minimizing the overall impact on blood sugar levels. Furthermore, employing heart-healthy oils like olive or avocado oil for air-frying delivers necessary fats to your diet.

4. **Maillard Reaction and Taste Development:** The Maillard reaction is a complicated chemical process that happens when

food browns while cooking, imparting taste and aroma. While this response is favorable for flavor, it may alter the item's glycemic index.

Air-frying generates the Maillard reaction without the excessive browning and charring that happen with other high-temperature cooking techniques. This results in tasty meals that do not have a high blood sugar level.

5. **Portion Control and Meal Composition:** Air-frying helps with portion control as it requires less oil while preserving flavor. This component is crucial for maintaining blood sugar levels, as portion sizes directly impact the quantity of carbs and other nutrients taken.

Air-frying enables you to enjoy great meals without the need for huge amounts, which helps to improve blood sugar management. Knowing the complexities of how cooking techniques impact blood sugar, helps you make culinary choices that correspond with your health objectives.

Tips for Healthier Cooking with an Air Fryer

Unlocking the full power of your air fryer requires more than simply tossing food in the basket.

1. **Select the Right Air Fryer:** Choose an air fryer with changeable temperature settings for extra versatility while frying a range of meals. Consider a model with a big basket that allows for equal air circulation and can hold bulkier goods.

2. **Essential Tools and Accessories:** Invest in a kitchen thermometer to guarantee correct cooking temperatures and food safety. Use silicone or nonstick liners to minimize sticking and make cleaning easy. Experiment with devices such as skewers or racks to raise objects and promote air circulation.

3. **Mindful Oil Use:** Instead of soaking items in oil, use an oil sprayer to gently coat dishes with heart-healthy oils such as olive or avocado oil. Choose oils with high smoke points to prevent the development of hazardous chemicals during the air-frying process.

4. **Preheat when necessary:** Preheating is typically not necessary for air-frying, yet it could be useful in specific recipes. Preheat for a few minutes before preparing products that require a crisp exterior.

5. **Crisping techniques:** To produce a golden brown crispiness, pat dry materials before air-frying to eliminate unnecessary moisture. Try a tiny coating of whole-grain breadcrumbs or crushed almonds for increased texture without sacrificing nutrients.

6. **Batch cooking:** To guarantee even cooking, avoid overloading the air fryer basket. Cook food in batches, enabling hot air to flow around each item.

7. **Temperature and cooking time:** Refer to your air fryer's guidelines for suggested temperature settings and cooking times, and modify as required according to your preferences. Flip or shake the basket periodically during cooking to achieve consistent crispness.

8. **Experiment with seasoning:** Experiment with herbs, spices, and citrus zest to improve taste without adding sugar or salt.

Create unique spice combinations to give a personal touch to your food.

9. **Monitor food carefully:** Keep a tight check on the cooking process, particularly at the conclusion, to avoid overcooking and ensure that your dishes are precisely done.

10. **Ventilation and Smoke Management:** Ensure appropriate ventilation in your kitchen, particularly if you're using a high-temperature air fryer. Place the air fryer in an open location away from cabinetry to avoid smoke accumulation.

These tips will help you make the most of your air fryer while concentrating on health. From choosing the correct equipment to developing your culinary talents, you can confidently and effortlessly cook tasty, diabetic-friendly meals.

Chapter 1: Diabetic-Friendly Air Frying Basics

Choosing the Right Air Fryer for Your Needs

In the ever-changing world of kitchen equipment, selecting the greatest air fryer is more than simply a decision; it's a vow to a better and more tasty life. Let's look at the current variables to consider when picking the appropriate air fryer, a modern culinary companion adapted to your individual requirements.

1. **Air Fryer Types:** There are various air fryers on the market today, each with its own unique set of qualities. The typical basket-style air fryer is a popular option for its simplicity and convenience of operation.

The oven-style air fryer, on the other hand, fits smoothly into your kitchen, allowing for extra application beyond air frying. Understanding the distinctions between these kinds lets you make a pick that is suited for both your kitchen space and culinary tastes.

2. **Temperature Adjustments:** Look for an air fryer with changeable temperature settings that give the accuracy necessary for a range of recipes. The flexibility to fine-tune the temperature means that delicate components enjoy gentle cooking, whereas heartier foods may demand a more robust approach. This versatility is the key to releasing your air fryer's full culinary potential.

3. **Size Matters:** Consider the size of the air fryer in relation to your kitchen's dimensions. While a greater capacity allows for more complete meal preparation, it is crucial to establish a balance that corresponds to your available space.

An air fryer with a big basket enables controlled air circulation, resulting in consistently superb results without compromising your kitchen's productivity.

4. **Smart Features:** In the age of smart technology, you may acquire air fryers with new functionalities that enrich your cooking experience. From preset settings to smartphone

connections, these contemporary conveniences speed up the cooking process, delivering not only efficiency but also a touch of culinary expertise.

5. **User-Friendly Interface:** A user-friendly interface is vital for a seamless cooking experience. Temperature settings and cooking times are simply handled owing to easy controls and clear displays. As you begin on your air-frying journey, a well-designed interface ensures that your attention stays on preparing tasty, blood sugar-friendly meals.

Chapter 2: Breakfasts to Energize

Crispy Cinnamon Pancakes

Let us learn the secret behind Crispy Cinnamon Pancakes, a morning beauty. In this recipe, the air fryer turns ordinary pancake batter into a golden hug of morning comfort, blending the traditional warmth of cinnamon with a contemporary touch of crispiness.

Ingredients:

Pancake Batter: These pancakes are produced using a nutritious blend of flour, baking powder, and eggs. To add a nutritious boost, use whole-grain flour or alternative flours.

Milk or Milk Substitute: Select your chosen dairy or non-dairy milk to achieve the correct consistency in the pancake batter. Almond or oat milk lends a delicate nuttiness.

Cinnamon: The star of the show, cinnamon gives a fragrant warmth that enhances the taste profile. Its sweet and spicy undertones dance with each sip, producing a wonderful and fragrant experience.

Sweetener: A bit of sweetness, whether from ordinary sugar, honey, or a sugar alternative, improves the entire taste. Adjust the sweetness level to your tastes and dietary limits.

Vanilla Extract: A dash of vanilla extract provides depth and complexity, rounding out the taste profile and boosting overall richness.

Instructions:

Make the pancake batter:

- In a mixing basin, combine the flour, baking powder, eggs, milk, cinnamon, sugar, and vanilla extract.
- Whisk until a smooth batter develops, ensuring that the cinnamon is properly distributed.
- Preheat the air fryer.

- Set your air fryer to the optimal temperature for pancakes. Preheating enables a uniform and consistent cooking process.

Portion and cook: Using a ladle or measuring cup, pour pancake batter into the preheated air fryer basket. The heated air moving around each pancake gives it a delicious crispiness while preserving its soft core.

Cooking time should be modified as required to attain the proper amount of crispiness. The air fryer's efficiency provides for a faster cooking time than past processes.

Serve warm: Once the pancakes are golden and crispy, take them from the air fryer and serve warm. The scent of cinnamon will appeal to your senses, resulting in a delicious and diabetic-friendly breakfast experience.

Accompaniments: Top your crispy cinnamon pancakes with a mix of fresh berries or banana slices for a rush of natural sweetness and nutrition.

Nuts or Seeds: Add chopped nuts or seeds, such as almonds or chia seeds, for a delicious crunch and an extra dose of healthy fats.

Greek Yogurt: A dollop of Greek yogurt gives a creamy contrast to the crispy pancakes while also supplying protein to the meal.

Veggie-Packed Omelette Bites

The recipe for Veggie-Packed Omelette Bites emerges as a symphony of color, taste, and nutrient-rich delight. In this culinary masterpiece, the air fryer turns the basic omelette into useful and pleasant nibbles, delivering brightness and the positive energy required to start the day.

Ingredients:

- Eggs are the cornerstone of your omelette pieces and provide a high-quality source of protein, which is needed for a delicious and healthy morning.
- Choose a range of bright veggies for both taste and nutritional diversity.
- Bell peppers, tomatoes, spinach, and mushrooms are wonderful possibilities.
- Dice or slice the veggies finely to achieve a fair distribution.
- Cheese (optional)
- For extra richness and taste, try inserting a tiny bit of your favorite cheese. Choose varieties with rich tastes to make each mouthful memorable.
- **Herbs and Spices:** Add a sprinkling of fresh herbs like parsley or chives to improve the flavor profile.
- Seasonings like salt, pepper, and a dusting of garlic powder lend to the overall savory flavor.

Instructions:

Prepare the vegetable blend:

- In a bowl, combine the chopped veggies, ensuring a balanced blend of colors and textures. This combination not only adds to the visual beauty of your omelette portions, but it also supplies a varied spectrum of nutrients.

- **Whisk the eggs:** In a separate dish, beat the eggs until fully blended. Consider using egg whites or a mix of whole eggs and egg whites to minimize cholesterol while maintaining protein levels.

- **Season and combine:** Add the vegetable combination to the beaten eggs, along with the herbs, spices, and cheese, if preferred. Gently fold the ingredients together to produce a homogenous distribution.

- **Warm the Air Fryer:** Set your air fryer to the optimum temperature for eggs or omelettes and let it warm for the best frying results.

- **Portion and cook:** Divide the egg and vegetable mixture among the portions of a silicone mold or individual muffin cups. Put the molds or cups in the preheated air fryer basket.

- **Monitor and alter:** Keep a watchful eye on the cooking process and change the time as required to reach the appropriate amount of firmness. The air fryer's efficiency allows for exact control of the cooking duration.
- **Serve Warm:** Once the veggie-packed omelet bites are golden and fully cooked, take them from the air fryer. Allow them to cool momentarily before serving.

Accompaniments:

- **Avocado Slices:** Creamy avocado slices add richness to your omelette sections while offering healthy fats and a pleasant texture.
- **Salsa or Hot Sauce:** A dollop of fresh salsa or a sprinkle of hot sauce delivers a spicy kick to your taste receptors while complementing the savory tastes of the omelette portions.

- **Whole-grain bread:** For a healthy and balanced breakfast, serve your omelette bits with a side of whole-grain bread.

Almond Flour Waffles with Compote

Ingredients:

For the almond flour waffles:

Almond Flour: A nutrient-dense alternative to conventional flour, almond flour has a delightful nuttiness while still carrying protein and healthy fats.

Eggs: Eggs offer a protein boost and add to the structure and richness of the waffles.

Milk or Milk Substitute: Select your chosen dairy or non-dairy milk to acquire the required consistency. Almond milk complements the almond flour, giving it a nutty taste.

Sweetener: Use a sugar substitute or sweetener of your choosing to offer a touch of sweetness without boosting blood glucose levels.

Vanilla Extract: A dab of vanilla extract adds warmth and richness to the waffle batter, boosting its overall taste profile.

For Berry Compote

Mixed Berries: A beautiful combination of fresh or frozen berries—strawberries, blueberries, and raspberries—provides natural sweetness and a boost of antioxidants.

Sugar: To balance the acidity of the berries, add a tiny bit of sugar to taste.

Lemon Juice: A dab of lemon juice adds acidity and brightens the berry compote.

Instructions:

For the almond flour waffles: In a mixing dish, combine the almond flour, eggs, milk, sweetener, and vanilla extract. Whisk until a smooth batter develops.

Warm the Air Fryer: Preheat your air fryer to the optimal temperature for waffles, then leave it to warm for a homogenous frying operation.

Cook the waffles. Pour parts of the batter into the preheated air fryer basket. Cook the waffles until they are golden and crispy. Adjust the cooking time as required to attain the right amount of crispiness. The almond flour waffles will have a wonderful nutty scent.

For Berry Compote:

Ingredients: In a saucepan, combine the mixed berries, sugar, and lemon juice. Cook over medium heat until the berries have broken down and the mixture thickens into a compote.

Adjust Sweetness: Taste the compote and adjust the sweetness as required. The natural sugars in the berries add to their overall sweetness.

Place the almond flour waffles and liberally top with the warm berry compote. The contrast between crispy waffles and strawberry compote produces a delightful texture and taste experience.

Optional decorations include slivered almonds or powdered sugar for an extra touch of elegance and texture.

Chapter 3: Appetizers and Snacks

Zesty Guacamole Stuffed Mushrooms

Ingredients:

The earthy receptacles create a fantastic backdrop for the tasty guacamole. Choose mushrooms with firm tops for a simple filling.

Guacamole: Avocado is the star of the show, supported by chopped tomatoes, red onion, cilantro, lime juice, and a touch of salt. Guacamole provides smoothness and a zesty taste to the mushrooms.

Garlic: Freshly minced garlic provides the filling with an aromatic richness that enriches the overall savory taste.

Lime Juice: A dash of lime juice not only gives a tangy flavor to the guacamole but also helps avoid browning.

Salt and Pepper: Season to taste, combining the avocado's richness with the savory tones of salt and the warmth of black pepper. Optional garnishes include fresh cilantro or a sprinkling of chili flakes for an added blast of flavor and visual appeal.

Instructions:

- Prepare the mushrooms.
- Clean the mushrooms and carefully remove the stems, leaving a hollow for the guacamole filling.
- Place the mushrooms in an air fryer basket.

Make the guacamole:

Mash ripe avocados in a bowl, then add chopped tomatoes, red onion, minced garlic, cilantro, lime juice, salt, and pepper. Mix until the guacamole has a smooth and balanced consistency.

Stuff the Mushrooms: Spoon the guacamole into the mushroom caps, ensuring uniform distribution. The air fryer's strong heat will cook the mushrooms to perfection while keeping the guacamole's freshness.

Warm the Air Fryer: Set the air fryer to the ideal temperature for filled mushrooms and leave it to warm for the best results. Air fry to perfection: Place the filled mushrooms in a hot air fryer and cook until soft and the guacamole filling has warmed slightly. The air fryer offers the ultimate blend of delicate mushrooms and creamy guacamole.

Optional garnish: To increase taste and visual appeal, add fresh cilantro or chili flakes over the packed mushrooms.

Serve Warm: Place the Zesty Guacamole Stuffed

Mushrooms on a dish and serve warm. The brilliant colors and spicy perfume will encourage your visitors to try this tasty snack.

Pairing Suggestions:

Salsa Fresca: Serve the filled mushrooms with a side of fresh salsa for an added blast of acidity and flavor.

Lime Wedges: Serve lime wedges on the side so that visitors may modify the zesty tones of the guacamole to their preference..

Spiced Chickpea Snack Mix

In this air-fried meal, the air fryer takes center stage, infusing the chickpeas with a harmonizing combination of spices, resulting in a snack that is not only tasty but also conforms to diabetic-friendly principles.

Ingredients: Canned chickpeas comprise the snack mix's basis, delivering protein and fiber.

Olive Oil: A drizzle of heart-healthy olive oil improves the crunchiness of the chickpeas while imparting a subtle richness.

Spice Blend: A mixture of spices, such as cumin, paprika, garlic powder, and cayenne pepper, makes a delicious and savory covering for the chickpeas.

Salt and pepper: To taste, balance the spices and enhance the overall savory flavor of the snack mix. Consider incorporating additional ingredients such as roasted nuts, seeds, or dry herbs to add layers of texture and taste.

Instructions:

Prepare the chickpeas. Drain and rinse the canned chickpeas thoroughly. To eliminate any excess moisture, blot them dry with a clean kitchen towel or paper towel.

Seasoning Mix: In a bowl, add olive oil, spice mix, salt, and pepper. Stir thoroughly to produce a cohesive spice combination.

Coat the chickpeas: Combine the dry chickpeas with the spice mixture, ensuring they are thoroughly coated. The spices will attach to the chickpeas, forming a lovely crust during the air-frying process.

Preheat the Air Fryer: Set the air fryer to the optimum temperature for roasting chickpeas and allow it to preheat for the best results.

Air fry to perfection: Spread the seasoned chickpeas evenly in the air fryer basket to allow for optimal air circulation. Air-fry the chickpeas till brown and crispy, shaking the basket occasionally to ensure even frying.

Cool and Enjoy: Once completed, leave the spiced chickpea snack mix to cool for a few minutes. The chickpeas will continue to crisp during this time. Place the snack mix on a platter and serve it at room temperature.

Variations and serving suggestions:

Trail Mix Addition: For a savory-sweet trail mix, combine the spiced chickpeas with a selection of nuts, seeds, and dried fruit.

Yogurt Dip: For a refreshing contrast, serve the Spiced

Chickpea Snack Mix with a side of Greek yogurt dip seasoned with herbs and lemon juice.

Air-Fried Buffalo Cauliflower Bites

Ingredients:

Cauliflower Florets: On the meal's solid basis, cauliflower florets give a great texture that absorbs the powerful Buffalo sauce.

Buffalo Sauce: a mixture of hot sauce, melted butter or a butter replacement, and a splash of vinegar that gives the famed spicy and tangy Buffalo taste.

Olive Oil: A drizzle of olive oil improves the crispiness of the cauliflower portions while imparting a feeling of richness.

Garlic Powder and Onion Powder: These delightful components enrich the complete taste profile, complementing the fiery buffalo sauce.

Salt and pepper: to taste, balancing the flavors and giving a tiny spice to the cauliflower.

Garnish: Fresh parsley or chives may be sprinkled on top for a blast of flavor and visual appeal.

Instructions: Prepare the cauliflower. Wash and dry the cauliflower carefully. Cut into bite-sized florets to ensure consistent cooking.

Create the Buffalo Sauce: In a bowl, add the hot sauce, melted butter or butter replacement, vinegar, garlic powder, onion powder, salt, and pepper. Whisk together the ingredients until they produce a cohesive and hot Buffalo sauce.

Coat the cauliflower: Drizzle olive oil over the cauliflower florets and toss until evenly coated. Toss the cauliflower again with the Buffalo sauce, making sure to cover each floret thoroughly.

Warm the Air Fryer: Set the air fryer to the correct temperature for roasting vegetables and allow it to warm for the best results. **Air Fry to Perfection:** Spread the buffalo-coated cauliflower florets evenly in the air fryer basket to allow for optimum air circulation. Air fry until the cauliflower is golden brown and crispy, regularly shaking the basket to ensure even grilling. **Garnish and serve:** When completed, move the air-fried Buffalo Cauliflower Bites to a serving platter. Garnish with fresh parsley or chives for added taste and visual appeal.

Serve with Dipping Sauce: For an extra layer of indulgence, top the cauliflower pieces with a cold dipping sauce like ranch or blue cheese dressing.

Serving suggestions: Serve the air-fried buffalo cauliflower bites with traditional celery and carrot sticks for a refreshing and crisp contrast. A dish of Greek yogurt or a yogurt-based dip could help to cool down the heat from the Buffalo sauce.

This dinner demonstrates cauliflower's flexibility, delivering a crispy and tasty alternative to typical Buffalo wings. Whether savored as a solo snack or as a crowd-pleasing appetizer, each bite illustrates the satisfaction of robust tastes and health-conscious enjoyment.

Chapter 4: Wholesome Main Dishes

Herb-Roasted Chicken Thighs

In this air-fried delight, the air fryer performs the role of a maestro, converting ordinary chicken thighs into an exquisite delicacy filled with herb richness.

Ingredients:

Chicken Thighs: The chicken thighs offer a juicy and tasty foundation for the herb-roasting procedure.

Fresh Herbs: Fresh herbs such as rosemary, thyme, and oregano lend a wonderful scent to the meal, infusing the chicken with layers of exquisite flavor.

Garlic: Freshly minced garlic provides depth and richness, complementing the herbs and increasing the overall savory taste. A drizzle of olive oil improves the crispiness of the chicken skin while infusing it with a dash of healthy fats.

Lemon Zest: Lemon zest lends a zesty sharpness to the herb-roasted chicken, increasing its taste and adding a refreshing touch.

Salt and pepper: to taste, boost overall seasoning, and offer a well-balanced flavor profile.

Instructions: Prepare the chicken thighs. Pat the chicken thighs dry with a paper towel to eliminate any excess moisture. This strategy assures a crispy exterior throughout the air-frying procedure.

Make the herb marinade: In a bowl, mix the minced garlic, finely chopped fresh herbs, olive oil, lemon zest, salt, and pepper. Stir the ingredients together to produce a cohesive herb marinade.

Coat the Chicken: Generously coat each chicken thigh with the herb marinade, ensuring that the mixture is uniformly spread on both sides. Allow the chicken to marinate for at least 15–30 minutes so that the flavors may combine.

Warm the Air Fryer: Set the air fryer to the optimum temperature for roasting chicken and allow it to warm up for maximum cooking results.

Air Fry to Perfection: Place the herb-coated chicken thighs in the preheated air fryer basket in a single layer to achieve equal cooking. Air-fry the chicken thighs until they have a golden brown exterior and a juicy, tender interior.

Rest and Serve: Let the herb-roasted chicken thighs rest for a few minutes before serving. This rest interval helps the fluids redistribute, resulting in a succulent and enjoyable eating experience.

Pairing Suggestions:

Roasted veggies: For a substantial and healthy supper, pair the herb-roasted chicken thighs with air-fried or oven-roasted vegetables.

Herb-Infused Quinoa or Brown Rice: Serve the chicken with a side of herb-infused quinoa or brown rice to enhance the taste and provide nutritional benefits.

Mediterranean Turkey Burgers

Ingredients:

Ground Turkey: These burgers are produced with lean ground turkey, which offers a protein-rich and low-fat alternative to regular beef patties.

Mediterranean Herb Blend: A blend of dried oregano, basil, thyme, and rosemary gives the burgers a Mediterranean flavor, infusing them with fragrant and savory undertones.

Feta Cheese: Crumbled feta cheese offers a creamy texture and acidic taste that complements the Mediterranean herb mix.

Sun-Dried Tomatoes: Finely chopped sun-dried tomatoes offer a rush of sweetness and umami to the turkey burgers, boosting their overall taste profile.

Garlic: Freshly minced garlic enhances the exquisite aromas and adds depth to the Mediterranean-inspired hamburgers.

Egg: A beaten egg functions as a binding agent, ensuring that the burgers remain together throughout cooking.

Salt and pepper: to taste, harmonizing tastes and enhancing the overall seasoning.

Instructions:

Make the Turkey Burger Mixture: In a large mixing bowl, combine ground turkey, the Mediterranean herb blend, crumbled feta cheese, chopped sun-dried tomatoes, minced garlic, beaten egg, and salt and pepper. Mix the components until entirely integrated, resulting in a homogenous dispersion of tastes.

Shape the Patties: Divide the turkey mixture into equal quantities and make hamburger patties. The air fryer's efficacy assures consistent frying, enabling the patties to acquire a golden exterior while keeping them moist and tasty inside.

Warm the Air Fryer: Preheat the air fryer to the temperature specified for frying turkey burgers, then leave it to warm for optimal results.

Air fry to perfection: Place the formed turkey patties in the preheated air fryer basket, stacking them in a single layer.

Air-fry the burgers until they have a golden brown coating on the surface and are totally cooked on the inside.

Rest and Assemble: Let the Mediterranean Turkey Burgers rest for a few minutes before placing them on whole-grain buns. The resting phase enables the fluids to redistribute, resulting in a juicy and pleasurable bite.

Topping and Serving Suggestions: Drizzle or spread a dollop of tzatziki sauce on top of each burger for a cold and tangy kick. Top the burgers with a handful of fresh greens, like arugula or spinach, for extra crunch and nutrition.

Sliced Cucumber and Red Onion: For a burst of freshness and texture, add thin slices of cucumber and red onion to your Mediterranean cuisine.

Lemon Garlic Shrimp Skewers with Quinoa

Ingredients:

Shrimp: Fresh or frozen shrimp serve as the protein-rich foundation for this dish, making it both scrumptious and easy to make.

Lemon Zest and Juice: Freshly grated lemon zest and juice provide a bright citrus taste to the shrimp and quinoa.

Garlic: Minced garlic adds aromatic richness to the shrimp and quinoa, increasing their savory flavor.

Olive Oil: A drizzle of heart-healthy olive oil offers moisture to the food and improves its flavor.

Quinoa: Quinoa is a nutrient-dense grain that has a delicious nutty flavor and texture.

Fresh Parsley: Chopped fresh parsley offers a burst of freshness and color to your meal. Salt and pepper to taste, ensuring that the shrimp and quinoa are well-balanced in flavor.

Instructions: Prepare the shrimp. In a bowl, combine the shrimp, lemon zest, lemon juice, minced garlic, olive oil, salt, and pepper. Toss the items until the shrimp are well coated in the delicious marinade. Allow them to marinate for a while to absorb the scents.

Thread the Skewers: Thread the marinated shrimp onto skewers in a uniform distribution to ensure even cooking. The air fryer will cook the skewers thoroughly, resulting in a lovely char and flavor.

Warm the Air Fryer: Set the air fryer to the right temperature for frying shrimp skewers, then let it warm for maximum results.

Air fry to perfection: Place the shrimp skewers in the preheated air fryer basket, distributing them evenly for consistent cooking. Air-fry the shrimp until they have a golden exterior and are totally done.

Prepare the Quinoa: While the shrimp are air-frying, prepare the quinoa according to package directions. Quinoa supplies a protein- and fiber-rich supplement to the prawns. Assemble and serve the lemon-garlic shrimp skewers on a bed of cooked quinoa. Garnish with chopped fresh parsley for a bright accent.

Serving suggestions:

Lemon Wedges: Serve the meal with extra lemon wedges on the side, allowing diners to pour fresh lemon juice over the shrimp for a burst of zesty flavor.

Steamed vegetables: Serve with the shrimp skewers and quinoa to offer color, nutrition, and a diversity of textures.

Chapter 5: Vibrant Vegetarian Delights

Portobello Mushroom Fajitas

Ingredients:

Portobello Mushrooms: These meaty mushrooms are the centerpiece of the recipe, providing a deep and powerful base for the fajitas.

Bell Peppers: Sliced bell peppers give a variety of hues and a sweet, crisp texture to the fajitas. Thinly sliced red onion adds a little pungency and enriches the overall taste profile. The trademark fajita flavor is formed by blending spices such as cumin, chili powder, paprika, garlic powder, and oregano, which infuse the mushrooms and veggies with robust and delicious overtones.

Olive Oil: A dusting of olive oil enriches the cooking process, giving the fajitas a lovely sear and richness.

Lime Juice: Freshly squeezed lime juice provides tanginess and lemony brightness to the fajitas, improving their flavors.

Tortillas: Use whole-grain or corn tortillas to wrap the delicious mushroom and veggie combo.

Instructions:

Prepare the Portobello mushrooms: Clean the portobello mushrooms and remove their stems. Slice the caps into thin strips to simulate the texture of classic fajita meat.

Make the Fajita combine: In a bowl, combine the sliced Portobello mushrooms, bell peppers, and red onion with olive oil, fajita spice, and freshly squeezed lime juice. Ensure that the spices are uniformly covered on the veggies.

Warm the Air Fryer: To obtain the best results, set the air fryer to the desired temperature for frying vegetables and let it warm.

Air Fry to Perfection: Place the seasoned Portobello mushroom and vegetable combination in the preheated air fryer basket, spreading them out for even cooking. Air fry until the veggies have a sear and the mushrooms are soft and flavorful.

Warm the Tortillas: In the final minutes of air-frying, warm the tortillas in the air fryer or another way until they are malleable for wrapping. Assemble the Fajitas. Spoon the air-fried Portobello mushroom and veggie mixture onto the heated tortillas. Garnish with extra lime wedges, cilantro, or other favorite toppings.

Serving suggestions: Guacamole and Salsa: For an added rich and fresh taste, serve the Portobello Mushroom Fajitas with guacamole and salsa on the side.

Greek Yogurt or Sour Cream: A dollop of Greek yogurt or sour cream gives a relaxing counterpoint to the hot flavors of the fajitas. Sprinkle a piece of shredded cheese over the filling for a melty and delectable finish.

Sweet Potato and Black Bean Enchiladas

Ingredients:

Sweet potatoes: These vibrant orange tubers add a natural sweetness and nutritional boost to the enchiladas, giving them a healthier alternative to typical fillings.

Black Beans: The protein-rich black beans offer heartiness and a deep earthy flavor to the enchilada filling.

Corn Tortillas: Soft corn tortillas serve as an ideal vessel for wrapping the sweet potato and black bean mixture, providing a gluten-free alternative for individuals with dietary requirements.

Enchilada Sauce: A spicy and tasty enchilada sauce ties the components together, giving each mouthful a powerful and savory taste.

Cumin, Chili Powder, and Cilantro: This spice combination, when blended with fresh cilantro, enriches the Mexican-inspired taste profile, delivering a harmonic balance of warmth and freshness.

Cheese (optional): Shredded cheese may be added for an additional layer of richness and delight.

Instructions: Prepare the filling. Roast or air-fry chopped sweet potatoes until soft and lightly browned. In a bowl, mix the roasted sweet potatoes, black beans, cumin, chili powder, and chopped cilantro. Mix thoroughly to achieve a tasty and balanced filling.

Warm the Tortillas: Heat the corn tortillas swiftly, either in the air fryer or another way, to make them flexible for rolling.

Assemble the enchiladas: Spread the sweet potato and black bean mixture over each tortilla and roll firmly, placing the seam side down in a baking dish.

Pour Enchilada Sauce: Pour the enchilada sauce over the rolled tortillas, ensuring they are fully covered. Bake or air-fry the enchiladas until they're thoroughly done and the sauce is bubbling.

Optional: Sprinkle shredded cheese on top in the final few minutes of cooking for a melty finish.

Garnish and serve: Remove the enchiladas from the oven or air fryer and sprinkle with additional cilantro. Serve them with your choice of toppings, such as chopped avocado, Greek yogurt, or salsa.

Serving suggestions:

Avocado Slices: Serve slices of creamy avocado on the side to create a refreshing and buttery contrast to the scorching enchiladas.

Lime Wedges: Serve the enchiladas with lime wedges for a refreshing squeeze. Serve the enchiladas with a side salad of mixed greens, cherry tomatoes, and a light vinaigrette for a refreshing variation.

Crispy Tofu Stir-Fry

Ingredients:

Firm Tofu: Cubes of firm tofu serve as the protein-packed centerpiece of this stir-fry, offering a neutral canvas for the meal's intense flavors.

Colorful vegetables: bell peppers, broccoli, carrots, and snap peas add visual appeal and a diversity of textures to the stir-fry. Soy sauce, sesame oil, and fresh ginger infuse the stir-fry with salty, nutty, and fragrant ingredients, resulting in a rich taste profile.

Garlic and Green Onions: Minced garlic and sliced green onions offer fragrant richness and freshness to the meal.

Cornstarch: Coating the tofu cubes with cornstarch before air-frying gives them a crunchy texture that contrasts beautifully with the delicate center. Toasted sesame seeds (optional) may be sprinkled on top for a nutty and visually pleasing garnish.

Instructions: Prepare the tofu: Drain and press the firm tofu to eliminate extra moisture. Cut it into bite-sized pieces and cover them evenly with cornstarch. Air-fry the tofu. Preheat the air fryer and cook the cornstarch-coated tofu cubes until golden and crispy. This process ensures that the tofu becomes the star, with a delightful crunch.

Prepare the stir-fry sauce: Combine soy sauce, sesame oil, and chopped ginger in a bowl to produce a fragrant stir-fry sauce. Stir-fry the veggies. In a wok or pan, sauté the multicolored vegetables until crisp-tender. To add a fragrant touch, incorporate minced garlic and chopped green onions.

Combine and Toss: When the veggies are cooked, add the air-fried crispy tofu to the pan. Pour the stir-fry sauce over the tofu and veggies, turning to cover evenly. Garnish and serve with toasted sesame seeds for extra taste and visual appeal. Serve the crispy tofu stir-fry over steaming rice or noodles.

Serving suggestions: Serve the stir-fry over a bed of healthy brown rice or quinoa for a satisfying and nutritious meal. Garnish the meal with chili flakes or a sprinkling of Sriracha for those who want a spicy kick. Garnish with fresh cilantro leaves for a blast of freshness and herbal flavor.

Chapter 6: Sides That Satisfy

Garlic Parmesan Brussels Sprouts

Grated Parmesan cheese provides a savory and rich flavor to the air-fried Brussels sprouts, resulting in a delightful crust.

Garlic: Freshly minced garlic provides aromatic depth to the sprouts and enriches the overall savory taste of the dish. A tiny bit of high-quality olive oil delivers a healthy dose of fat while also making the food crispier. Season to taste with salt and pepper, ensuring that the spiciness is balanced and brings out the characteristics of the Brussels sprouts.

Instructions: First things first, prepare your Brussels sprouts by halving them and removing the stems. Ensure that they are dry, as this encourages greater caramelization during the air-frying process.

Make the Parmesan coating: In a bowl, mix the split Brussels sprouts, grated Parmesan cheese, chopped garlic, olive oil, salt, and pepper. Toss the ingredients until the sprouts are fully covered in the delicious mix.

Warm the Air Fryer: Preheat the air fryer to the optimum temperature for roasting vegetables, then allow it to warm for ideal cooking conditions.

Air fry to perfection: Place the coated Brussels sprouts in the preheated air fryer basket, spreading them evenly to guarantee consistent cooking. Air-fry the Brussels sprouts until they are golden brown on the outside and gently caramelized on the interior.

Serve immediately: Once the garlic parmesan Brussels sprouts have been air-fried to perfection, transfer them to a serving dish. Serve immediately, allowing the sprouts to achieve their pinnacle of crispness.

Garnish and serving suggestions: Garnish the garlic Parmesan Brussels sprouts with chopped fresh herbs like parsley or chives for a blast of freshness.

Lemon Wedges: Serve the sprouts with lemon wedges on the side, enabling guests to pour fresh lemon juice over the caramelized delicacies for a zesty kick.

Additional Parmesan: For those who want an additional layer of cheesy delight, throw a little more grated Parmesan on top before serving.

Cauliflower Mash with Chives

Cauliflower: Cauliflower has a mild taste and velvety texture, giving it a low-carb alternative to typical mashed potatoes.

Chives: Fresh chives offer a subtle onion flavor and a vivid green color to the cauliflower mash, boosting both its look and taste.

Butter: A tiny bit of butter gives richness and a nice, velvety texture to the mash.

Garlic: Minced garlic improves the taste profile of the mash, providing a mild savory note.

Chicken or vegetable broth (optional): Broth may be added for taste and to change the consistency of the cauliflower mash.

Salt and pepper: Season to taste, producing a well-balanced seasoning that enhances the cauliflower's intrinsic characteristics.

Instructions:

Prepare the cauliflower: Cut the cauliflower into florets of equivalent size for consistent cooking. Steam or boil the cauliflower until fork-tender. Alternatively, air-fry the cauliflower to obtain a roasted taste and improved sweetness.

Air Fry or Roast: Preheat the air fryer to a suitable temperature for roasting veggies. Toss the cauliflower florets with olive oil, salt, and pepper before air-frying until golden brown.

Blend or Mash: Place the cooked cauliflower in a food processor or use a hand masher to blend until smooth. To attain the proper consistency, mix in butter, minced garlic, and, if preferred, a dash of chicken or vegetable stock. Season and decorate the cauliflower mash with salt and pepper as desired. Fold in the fresh chives, saving some for decoration.

Serve Warm: Transfer the Cauliflower Mash with Chives to a serving dish and sprinkle with extra chopped chives. Serve the mash warm as a delightful and healthy alternative to typical mashed potatoes.

Serving suggestions:

Grated Parmesan: Before serving, put a tiny quantity of grated Parmesan on top for an extra layer of wonderful richness.

Sour Cream or Greek Yogurt: To add creaminess, top the cauliflower mash with a dollop of sour cream or Greek yogurt. Garnish with toasted, slivered almonds for a great crunch and nutty taste.

Rosemary Roasted Sweet Potatoes

Sweet Potatoes: The vibrant orange flesh of sweet potatoes is the focus of this dish, delivering natural sweetness and a wealth of nutrients.

Fresh Rosemary: Fragrant rosemary sprigs infuse the sweet potatoes with earthy and piney undertones, boosting the overall taste profile. A spray of quality olive oil enriches the taste and crispy texture of the roasted sweet potatoes.

Garlic (optional): For those who wish to add extra flavor to their sweet potatoes, minced garlic may be added. Salt and pepper to taste, for a well-balanced spice that brings out the inherent flavors of the sweet potatoes.

Instructions: Prepare the sweet potatoes. Wash and peel the sweet potatoes before cutting them into uniform pieces. This promotes consistent cooking and a uniform texture.

Coat with Olive Oil and Seasonings: In a mixing bowl, combine the sweet potato cubes, olive oil, fresh rosemary leaves, chopped garlic (if using), salt, and pepper. Ensure that the sweet potatoes are uniformly covered in the fragrant mixture.

Warm the Air Fryer: Preheat the air fryer to the optimum temperature for roasting vegetables, then allow it to warm for ideal cooking conditions. Air fry to perfection: Arrange the seasoned sweet potato cubes in a single layer in the preheated air fryer basket. Air-fry the sweet potatoes until they have a golden brown surface and a soft, caramelized middle.

Garnish and Serve: Once the rosemary-roasted sweet potatoes have been air-fried to perfection, arrange them in a serving dish.

Garnish with extra-fresh rosemary sprigs for visual appeal.

Serving suggestions: Balsamic Glaze: Before serving, pour a balsamic glaze over the roasted sweet potatoes to provide a sweet and tart contrast. Crumble feta or goat cheese over the top for a creamy and wonderful topping.

Pomegranate Seeds: Sprinkle colorful pomegranate seeds over the meal to add a burst of freshness and color.

Chapter 7: Sensational Sauces and Dips

Sugar-Free BBQ Sauce

In this air-fried age, the air fryer performs a supporting role, ready to cover your favorite foods in the delicious enticement of sugar-free BBQ sauce.

Ingredients:

Tomato Paste: Tomato paste is a powerful basis for the sauce, offering a deep and concentrated tomato taste without the need for added sweeteners.

Apple Cider Vinegar: The tart acidity of apple cider vinegar enriches the entire taste profile while adding brightness to the sauce.

Liquid Smoke: A spray of liquid smoke produces a smokey smell evocative of traditional barbecue without depending on sweet additives. Dijon mustard delivers a powerful kick and contributes to the BBQ sauce's wide flavor profile. **Worcestershire Sauce:** This umami-rich sauce enriches the mixture by providing depth and flavor.

Garlic and onion powder: These fragrant powders give the sauce layers of great richness, improving its overall complexity.

Paprika and Cumin: The smokey spices of paprika and the earthy warmth of cumin improve the sauce's overall taste.

Cayenne Pepper (Optional): For those who desire a little heat, cayenne pepper may be added to taste.

Salt and pepper: to taste, for a well-balanced seasoning that enhances the smokey and savory tastes. Instructions:

Ingredients: In a saucepan, add tomato paste, apple cider vinegar, liquid smoke, Dijon mustard, Worcestershire sauce, garlic powder, onion powder, paprika, cumin, cayenne pepper (if preferred), salt, and pepper.

Simmer and blend: Cook the mixture over low heat, permitting the flavors to merge. For a smoother texture, mix the sauce using an immersion blender or transfer it to a normal blender. Blend until the appropriate consistency is attained.

Adjust and cool: Taste the sauce and adjust the spices as required. Allow the sugar-free BBQ sauce to cool to room temperature. Transfer the sauce to a tight jar and refrigerate until ready for use. Use it as a wonderful coating for air-fried dishes or as a dipping sauce.

Serving suggestions:

Air-Fried Chicken Wings: Drizzle sugar-free BBQ sauce over crispy air-fried chicken wings for a wonderful and guilt-free treat.

Grilled veggies: Use the sauce as a marinade or glaze over air-fried or grilled vegetables, giving them a savory and smokey taste.

Pulled Chicken or Pork: Combine the sugar-free BBQ sauce with shredded air-fried chicken or pork to produce a great sandwich or taco filler.

Greek Yogurt Ranch Dip

Ingredients:

Greek Yogurt: The star of the show, Greek yogurt offers a creamy and tangy basis for the dip while also offering a decent amount of protein.

Fresh Herbs (Dill, Chives, and Parsley): A combination of fresh herbs, such as dill, chives, and parsley, adds rich flavor and a burst of freshness to the dip.

Garlic: Minced garlic adds flavor to the ranch dip, boosting its overall depth.

Lemon Juice: Fresh lemon juice gives a tangy and zesty freshness that balances out the richness of the Greek yogurt.

Dijon Mustard: Dijon mustard provides a little spice and depth of flavor to the dip.

Onion Powder: Onion powder delivers a modest onion taste without the texture of raw onions. Salt and pepper: to taste, for a well-balanced flavor that matches the richness of the Greek yogurt.

Instructions:

Prepare the herbs: Finely cut the fresh herbs, including dill, chives, and parsley, for a fine and uniform dispersion of tastes.

Ingredients: In a mixing bowl, combine Greek yogurt, garlic, herbs, lemon juice, Dijon mustard, onion powder, salt, and pepper. Mix the ingredients carefully to produce a uniform and creamy texture.

Chill and Let Flavors Melt: Cover the bowl and refrigerate the Greek Yogurt Ranch Dip for at least an hour to enable the flavors to blend and deepen. Taste the dip and adjust the seasoning as required, adding additional salt, pepper, or lemon juice to attain the desired taste profile.

Serve and enjoy: Once cooled, pour the Greek Yogurt Ranch Dip into a serving dish. Serve with your favorite air-fried foods, fresh veggies, or as a savory spice.

Serving suggestions:

Carrot and Celery Sticks: For a crisp and tasty snack, dip fresh carrot and celery sticks in Greek Yogurt Ranch Dip.

Air-Fried Chicken Tenders: For a delightful and guilt-free treat, cover crispy air-fried chicken tenders in this tangy and herb-infused dip. Serve with roasted potato wedges, which are a creamy and tasty alternative to typical dipping sauces.

Fresh Salsa with Avocado

Ingredients:

Tomatoes: Ripe and juicy tomatoes constitute the basis, offering a blast of freshness and a touch of sweetness.

Red onion: A finely sliced red onion offers a mild onion flavor and a brilliant flash of color to the salsa. Fresh cilantro, freshly chopped, lends an herbaceous and lemony element to the entire taste profile. Deseeded and thinly sliced jalapeño provides spiciness to contrast the sweetness of the tomatoes.

Lime Juice: Fresh lime juice provides a strong acidity that enriches the salsa.

Garlic: Minced garlic gives taste depth to the other fresh and vibrant components.

Avocado: Chop a creamy and ripe avocado to give the salsa a rich, velvety texture.

Salt and pepper: To taste, add a well-balanced seasoning that complements the inherent tastes of the components.

Instructions: Prepare the ingredients. Dice tomatoes, finely cut red onion, cilantro, jalapeño, and mince garlic. Peel, pit, and dice a ripe avocado. In a mixing dish, add diced tomatoes, red onion, cilantro, jalapeño, minced garlic, and avocado.

Add Lime Juice and Seasoning: Squeeze fresh lime juice evenly over the mixture. Add salt and pepper to taste, adjusting seasoning as required.

Gently mix: Gently blend the ingredients to ensure that the avocado is equally distributed without breaking its creamy smoothness. chill and let flavors melt. Cover the dish and refrigerate the fresh salsa with avocado for at least 30 minutes to permit the flavors to combine and enhance.

Adjust Seasoning: Before serving, taste the salsa and add extra lime juice, salt, or pepper to taste.

Serve and enjoy: Once cold, transfer the fresh salsa with avocado to a serving platter. Serve it as a bright topping for air-fried items, as a dip with tortilla chips, or as a refreshing side.

Serving suggestions:

Grilled Shrimp Tacos: Pour the fresh salsa with avocado over the grilled shrimp tacos for a blast of freshness and creaminess.

Air-Fried Tortilla Chips: Pair the salsa with homemade air-fried tortilla chips for a nutritious and tasty snack.

Crispy Chicken Tenders: Serve crispy air-fried chicken tenders with this salsa for a lovely and satisfying supper.

Chapter 8: Sweet Treats with a Healthy Twist

Air-Fried Apple Chips

Ingredients:

Apples: For a delicious blend of sweetness and bitterness, choose fresh and firm apples like Honeycrisp or Granny Smith.

Cinnamon: Ground cinnamon has a warm and fragrant flavor that enhances the natural sweetness of apples.

Optional: Sugar Substitute (Stevia, Erythritol): If desired, a tiny quantity of sugar substitute may be used to boost sweetness without adding extra sugar.

Instructions: Prepare the apples. Wash and slice the apples thinly, maintaining an identical thickness for uniform air frying. For uniform slices, try using a mandoline slicer.

Coat with Cinnamon: In a dish, toss the apple slices with ground cinnamon until uniformly covered. If using a sugar substitute, add it with the cinnamon for a hint of sweetness.

Preheat the Air Fryer: Set the air fryer to the appropriate temperature for dehydrating or roasting fruits.

Arrange on the Air Fryer Basket: Place the coated apple slices in a single layer on the air fryer basket, ensuring they do not overlap to facilitate equal air circulation. Air-fry the apple slices until crispy and golden brown, which normally takes 1 to 2 hours depending on their thickness.

Flip the slices halfway through cooking time to guarantee equal crispiness. Allow the apple chips to cool on a wire rack after air-frying them until they are ideally crispy. They will continue to crisp as they cool. Keep in an airtight container for ongoing eating.

Serving suggestions: Air-fried apple chips may be eaten plain or dipped for a naturally sweet and crispy snack. Dip them in a Greek yogurt-based dip or drizzle with some almond butter for added flavor. Apple chips may be blended with a variety of nuts and seeds to form a healthy and appetizing trail mix.

Ice Cream Topping: For a delightful and guilt-free dessert, scatter the apple chips over a scoop of vanilla sugar-free ice cream.

Dark Chocolate-Dipped Strawberries

Ingredients:

Fresh Strawberries: Choose ripe and firm strawberries with brilliant red colors to offer a delightful and juicy base for this wonderful meal.

Dark Chocolate: For a deep taste, use high-quality dark chocolate with at least 70% cocoa. If you prefer, pick sugar-free or low-sugar choices.

Extra Toppings: To boost the texture and taste, try adding chopped almonds, shredded coconut, or a sprinkle of sea salt.

Instructions:

Prepare the strawberries: Wash and thoroughly dry the strawberries, ensuring they are fully moisture-free to allow chocolate to cling.

Melt the Dark Chocolate: Break the dark chocolate into tiny pieces and melt in a double boiler or microwave, stirring regularly to produce a smooth consistency. Take care not to overheat the chocolate.

Dunk the Strawberries: Holding each strawberry by the stem, plunge it into the melting dark chocolate to achieve uniform coverage. Allow the extra chocolate to trickle off, or gently shake the strawberry to remove the excess coating.

Place on parcel paper: Place the chocolate-dipped strawberries on a pan lined with parchment paper, ensuring they don't touch to avoid sticking.

Optional Toppings: If preferred, add chopped almonds, shredded coconut, or sea salt over the chocolate-dipped strawberries before they firm.

Chill to Set: Refrigerate the tray of chocolate-dipped strawberries so that the chocolate may set and solidify. This normally takes roughly 30 minutes to an hour.

Serve and enjoy: Once the dark chocolate has completely solidified, arrange the strawberries on a dish. Serve and enjoy these delectable delights at once, or preserve them in the refrigerator for later.

Serving suggestions: Arrange the dark chocolate-dipped strawberries on an excellent dessert tray for a stylish display at parties or special events.

Dessert Skewers: Thread chocolate-dipped strawberries onto skewers for a quick and visually attractive way to consume this delectable delicacy.

Pair with red wine: Serve these lovely strawberries with a glass of red wine for a sumptuous and indulgent match.

Cinnamon Sugar Donut Holes

Ingredients: Choose all-purpose flour or almond flour for a normal or gluten-free choice. Baking powder offers the essential lift to make airy, fluffy donut holes. Salt enriches the overall taste by balancing the sweetness. Ground cinnamon fills the donut holes with a warm, fragrant scent. The egg gives structure and moisture to the dough. Milk provides richness and enhances the smooth texture of the donut holes.

Vanilla Extract: Adds a dash of vanilla flavor for depth. Unsweetened applesauce is a natural sweetener that helps with the moistness of the donut holes.

Butter or coconut oil: Provides a rich, buttery taste to the dough. Granulated sugar or a sugar substitute sweetens the dough.

For coating: Cover the newly made donut holes with granulated sugar or a sugar replacement. A delicious coating is formed by blending ground cinnamon and sugar.

Instructions: Make the dough. In a mixing basin, add flour, baking powder, salt, and powdered cinnamon. In a separate dish, mix the egg, milk, vanilla extract, applesauce, melted butter or coconut oil, and sugar.

Combine Wet and Dry Components: Gradually add the wet components to the dry, stirring just until incorporated. Be cautious not to overmix.

Donut Holes: To create the donut holes, form miniature dough balls using a little scoop or your hands. Preheat the air fryer. Set the air fryer to the appropriate temperature for baking or roasting. Air fry until golden brown. Place the produced donut holes in the air fryer basket, ensuring they do not overlap. Air-fry until golden brown and wonderfully done, which frequently takes 8–10 minutes.

Coating with Cinnamon Sugar: While the donut holes are still warm, carefully dip them into a mixture of granulated sugar (or sugar substitute) and ground cinnamon until uniformly coated.

Serve and enjoy. Place the cinnamon sugar donut holes on a serving plate and eat them warm.

Serving suggestions:

Coffee or Tea: Pair these Cinnamon Sugar Donut Holes with your favorite coffee or tea for a wonderful morning or afternoon snack.

Dipping Sauce: To enhance flavor, serve with sugar-free fruit preserves or a simple yogurt dip.

Ice Cream Topping: Top the donut holes with a tiny scoop of sugar-free vanilla ice cream.

Conclusion

This book is more than simply a compilation of recipes; it is a monument to the conviction that one may enjoy the delights of cooking while making responsible decisions that correspond to a diabetic-friendly lifestyle.

In our research, the air fryer emerged as a flexible partner, not only for making crispy treats but also for rewriting classics, experimenting with tastes, and presenting a healthier alternative to cherished recipes.

The recipes on these pages are more than simply a list of ingredients and directions; they are an invitation to embark on a culinary adventure that celebrates the delight of eating properly without sacrificing flavor.

From the savory joys of Diabetic-Friendly Air Frying Basics to the bright inventiveness of Sweet Treats with a Healthy Twist, each chapter offers up a new world of possibilities. We've witnessed the air fryer's power to convert everyday dishes into crispy masterpieces, learned the technique of producing guilt-free delights, and understood that health-conscious living can coexist with gourmet satisfaction.

But this conclusion is more than simply the end; it's the beginning of fresh knowledge, culinary confidence, and a road to a healthier and more tasty existence. As you leave these pages, may you be motivated to be creative in your kitchen, daring enough to experiment with conscious choices, and happy to relish each mouthful knowing that it feeds both body and spirit.

So here's to your culinary experiences, to the crispiness of air-fried marvels, and to the vivid tapestry of tastes that make every meal a feast. May your kitchen continue to be a haven of exploration, ingenuity, and, most importantly, sustenance that represents your dedication to living a diabetic-friendly, enjoyable life.

Until we meet again, happy cooking!